My Ultimate Mediterranean Se Diet Collection

Healthy & Fit with My Mediterranean Coooking Plan

Mateo Buscema

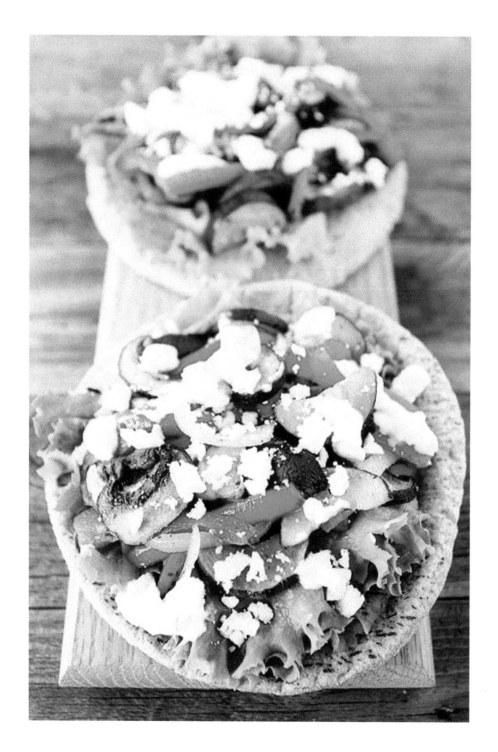

indirect, which are incurred as a result of the use of information contained within this document, including, but not limited to, — errors, omissions, or inaccuracies.

TABLE OF CONTENTS

Chickpea and spinach salad with avocado

This meal makes a staple diet in the Mediterranean countries with variety of vegetables and herbs to give it a maximum flavor for lunch and dinner.

Ingredients

- 1 avocado, sliced
- 1 pound of fresh spinach
- 1 red pepper, chopped
- 3 tomatoes, chopped
- 1 bunch of fresh cilantro, chopped
- Salt and pepper
- ½ cup of extra virgin olive oil
- 1 onion, sliced
- 1 pound of boiled or canned chickpeas
- Balsamic vinegar
- 1 cup of mushrooms, sliced

Directions

1. Together, put chickpeas with tomatoes, mushrooms, avocado, onion, red pepper, spinach, and cilantro in a mixing bowl.
2. Add salt and pepper to your liking.
3. Add olive oil together with the balsamic vinegar to taste.
4. Mix and serve.
5. Enjoy.

Spinach, chicken and feta salad

Ingredients

- 1 teaspoon of sugar
- 1 package of prewashed baby spinach
- 1 teaspoon of bottled minced garlic
- ½ teaspoon of salt
- 1 tablespoon of fresh lemon juice
- 1 teaspoon of Dijon mustard
- 1 teaspoon of olive oil
- ¼ cup of fat-free, chicken broth
- 1 can chickpeas drained
- 1 pound of skinless, boneless chicken breast
- ½ teaspoon of grated lemon rind
- ¼ teaspoon of black pepper
- Cooking spray
- 1 ½ cups of chopped red onion
- 1 tablespoon of balsamic vinegar
- 1 ¼ cups of pieces of yellow bell pepper
- ½ cup of crumbled feta cheese

Directions

1. Combine chicken broth, lemon rind, lemon juice, vinegar, sugar, garlic, dijon mustard, olive oil, and salt in a bowl and whisk.

2. Heat a large skillet coated after coating with cooking spray over medium-high heat.

3. Sprinkle chicken with black pepper.

4. Add chicken to pan let cook for 4 minutes, flip over.

5. Add onions and cook for 4 more minutes. Make sure to stir frequently.

6. Cut chicken into thick slices.

7. Combine chicken together with the onion, cheese, bell pepper, chickpeas, and spinach in a large bowl.

8. Drizzle with vinaigrette over salad and toss well.

9. Serve and enjoy.

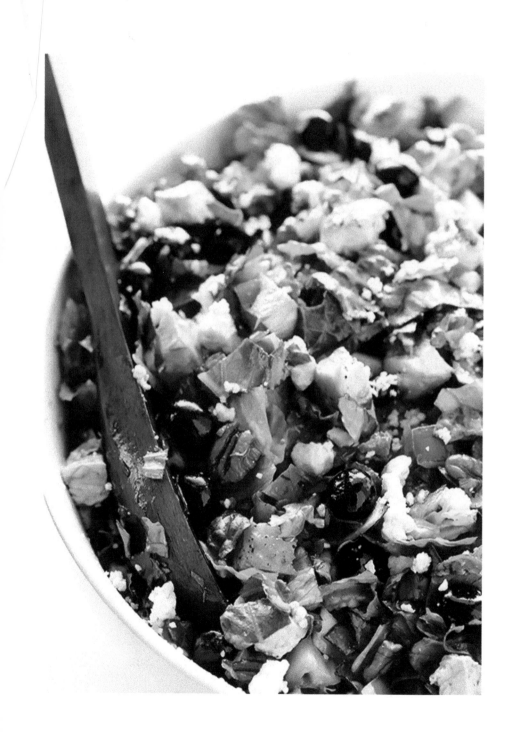

Mediterranean chicken salad pitas

No doubt everyone loves eating chicken; as such, this Mediterranean chicken salad pita comes in a new twist with greed thick yogurt.

It also has a rich flavor consistence.

Ingredients

- ½ Teaspoon of ground cumin
- 6 slices of tomato, cut in half
- 3 cups of chopped cooked chicken
- ½ cup of chopped pitted green olives
- Cup of plain whole-milk Greek yogurt
- ½ cup of diced red onion
- ¼ cup of chopped fresh cilantro
- 1 can of chickpeas, rinsed and drained
- 2 tablespoons of lemon juice
- 6 whole wheat pitas, cut in half
- Cup of chopped red bell pepper
- 12 bib lettuce leaves
- ¼ teaspoon of crushed red pepper

Directions

1. Combine the yogurt, lemon juice, cumin, and red pepper in a small mixing dish.

2. Combine chicken together with bell pepper, green olives, red onion, cilantro, and chickpeas in another separate small mixing dish.

3. Mix the two mixtures above and toss to coat.

4. Line each pita half with 1 lettuce leaf and 1 tomato piece.

5. Then, at least add ½ cup of chicken mixture to each pita half.

6. Serve and enjoy.

Halibut with lemon fennel salad

Ingredients

- 1 teaspoon of fresh thyme leaves
- 1 tablespoon of chopped flat-leaf parsley
- ½ teaspoon of salt
- 5 teaspoons of extra-virgin olive oil, divided
- 4 halibut fillets
- 2 garlic cloves, minced
- 2 cups of thinly sliced fennel bulb.
- ¼ cup of thinly vertically sliced red onion
- ¼ teaspoon of freshly ground black pepper
- 1 teaspoon of ground coriander
- ½ teaspoon of ground cumin
- 2 tablespoons of fresh lemon juice

Directions

1. In a small mixing bowl, combine coriander with salt, cumin, and black pepper.
2. Then, combine the spice mixture with oil and garlic in a small bowl.
3. Rub the garlic mixture evenly over fish.
4. Next, heat a large skillet over medium-high heat with oil to coat.

5. Add fish let cook for 5 minutes on every side.
6. Combine the balance of the spice mixture with oil balance and fennel bulb., and all ingredients in a medium bowl and toss.
7. Serve and enjoy salad with fish.

Pita salad with cucumber, fennel, and chicken

Ingredients

- 3 tablespoons of extra-virgin olive oil
- 2 cups of thinly sliced fennel bulb.
- ½ cucumber, halved lengthwise, sliced
- ½ cup of chopped fresh flat-leaf parsley
- 1 cup of shredded skinless, boneless rotisserie chicken breast
- ¼ teaspoon of black pepper, divided
- 2 pitas
- ¼ cup of fresh lemon juice
- 1 tablespoon of white wine vinegar
- ¼ cup of vertically sliced red onion
- ½ teaspoon of salt, divided
- ½ teaspoon of chopped fresh oregano

Directions

1. Firstly, preheat your oven to 350°F.
2. Organize your pitas on the baking sheet.
3. Bake for 12 minutes and toast well.
4. Let cool for 1 minute.

5. Then, break them into bite-sized pieces.
6. Combine pita pieces, fennel, together with chicken, parsley leaf, red onion, and cucumber in a dish.
7. Sprinkle with salt and pepper to season to taste.
8. Combine juice, oregano, vinegar, salt, and pepper in a bowl.
9. Whisk with oil.
10. Drizzle dressing over pita mixture and toss well.
11. Serve immediately and enjoy.

Orzo vegetable salad

Orzo vegetable salad's taste and delicacy is elevated with the tangy lemon dressing over chilled orzo and whole vegetables.

This vegetable recipe is a true Mediterranean Sea diet healthy for anyone and served along with any meal.

Ingredients

- ¼ teaspoon of pepper
- 3 plum of tomatoes, chopped
- 2 green onions, chopped
- 4 teaspoons of lemon juice
- 1 tablespoon minced fresh tarragon
- 2 teaspoons of grated lemon zest
- 1/3 cup of olive oil
- 1 cup of marinated artichoke hearts, chopped
- 1 cup of coarsely chopped fresh spinach
- ½ cup of crumbled feta cheese
- 2 teaspoons of rice vinegar
- 1 tablespoon of capers, drained
- ½ cup of uncooked orzo pasta
- ½ teaspoon of salt

Directions

1. Begin by cooking the orzo as per package Directions.
2. In a large bowl, combine artichokes, tomatoes, onions, spinach, cheese and capers.
3. In another small bowl, whisk all dressing ingredients.
4. Drain orzo and rinse.
5. Then add to vegetable mixture.
6. Pour dressing over salad, toss well.
7. Allow it to chill.
8. Serve and enjoy.

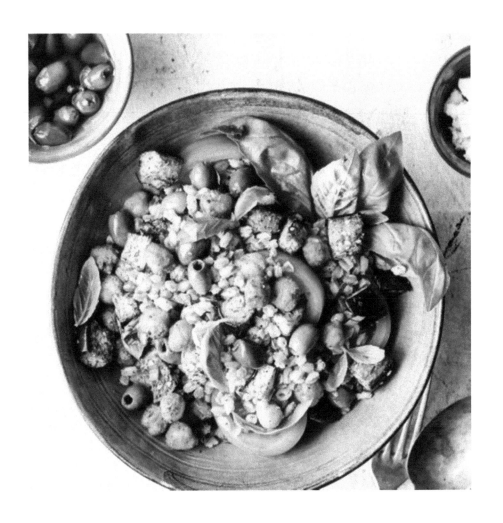

Balsamic cucumber salad

Ingredients

- ¾ cup crumbled reduced-fat feta cheese
- ½ cup balsamic vinaigrette
- 2 cups grape tomatoes, halved
- 1 large cucumber, halved and sliced
- 1 medium red onion, halved and sliced

Directions

1. In a large bowl, combine tomatoes, cucumber, and onion.
2. Add vinaigrette and toss to coat.
3. Cover properly and Refrigerate.
4. Stir in cheese before serving.
5. Serve and enjoy.

Greek couscous salad

These veggies are eaten raw as true Mediterranean Sea diet recipe; they are so hearty and delicious.

Ingredients

- ½ cup of olive oil
- ½ cup of crumbled feta cheese
- ¼ cup of lemon juice
- 1 teaspoon of adobo seasoning
- 1-¾ cups of uncooked whole wheat couscous
- 2 cups of grape tomatoes, halved
- 1 can of reduced-sodium chicken broth
- 1 cup of coarsely chopped fresh parsley
- 1-½ teaspoons of grated lemon zest
- ¼ teaspoon of salt
- 1 can of sliced ripe olives, drained
- 1 cucumber, halved lengthwise and sliced
- 4 green onions, chopped

Directions

1. In a large saucepan, bring broth to a boil.
2. Stir in couscous.

3. Remove from heat leave to settle covered to absorb the broth in 5 minutes.
4. Transfer to a large bowl let cool totally.
5. Whisk all dressing ingredients.
6. Add tomatoes, cucumber, olives, parsley, and green onions to couscous
7. Stir in the dressing.
8. Next, stir in cheese.
9. You can either serve immediately or refrigerate.
10. Serve cold and enjoy.

Mediterranean shrimp orzo salad

Trust me, this recipe will not fail to stand out on a buffet.

It is loaded with abundant shrimp, peppers, olives and artichoke hearts.

The components make a real Mediterranean Sea diet with variety of vegetables.

Ingredients

- ¾ cup of Greek vinaigrette
- 1/3 cup of chopped fresh dill
- ¾ pound of peeled and deveined cooked shrimp
- 1 cup of finely chopped green pepper
- 1 package of orzo pasta
- ¾ cup of finely chopped red onion
- ½ cup of pitted Greek olives
- 1 cup of finely chopped sweet red pepper
- ½ cup of minced fresh parsley
- 1 can of water-packed quartered artichoke hearts

Directions

1. Cook orzo as directed on the package.
2. Drain excess water when ready and rinse with cold water, drain again.
3. In a large bowl, combine orzo, vegetables, shrimp, olives, and herbs.
4. Add vinaigrette make sure to toss to coat.
5. Keep refrigerated when properly covered until serving.
6. Enjoy.

Arugula and wild rice salad

This recipe features toasted almond, feta, lemon dressing, dried cherries and of course arugula. It is gluten free and delicious for lunch and dinner.

Ingredients

- ½ cup of sliced almonds
- 5 ounces of arugula
- Freshly ground black pepper,
- 2 teaspoons of Dijon mustard
- ½ cup of coarsely chopped fresh basil
- 1 teaspoon of honey
- ½ cup of crumbled feta
- ½ teaspoon of olive oil
- 2 tablespoons of lemon juice
- 1 cup wild rice, rinsed
- 1 medium clove garlic
- ½ cup of dried tart cherries chopped
- ¼ teaspoon of sea salt

Directions

1. Bring a large pot of water to boil.

2. Add the rice cook for 20 – 35 minutes.
3. Remove, drain the rice and return to pot.
4. Cover let simmer for 10 minutes. Then uncover.
5. Warm 1 teaspoon of olive oil in a small skillet over medium temperature.
6. Add almonds and a pinch of salt let cook until golden and fragrant in 4 – 5 minutes.
7. In a small bowl, whisk dressing ingredients until blended.
8. Move the cooled rice to a large bowl.
9. Add arugula together with chopped basil, sour cherries, almonds, and feta.
10. Pour in the dressing, toss and season to taste with pepper.
11. Serve and enjoy.

Masala lentil salad with cumin roasted carrots

This recipe is protein rich form the lentils and fresh greens infused with vinaigrette.

A typical healthy Mediterranean Sea diet.

Ingredients

- 1 teaspoon garam masala
- 5 tablespoons extra-virgin olive oil
- ½ medium red onion, finely chopped
- 1 tablespoon maple syrup
- 1 ½ teaspoons ground cumin
- Salt and ground black pepper
- Toasted pumpkin seeds
- 2 tablespoons apple cider vinegar
- Ground black pepper
- 1 ½ pounds carrots, peeled and sliced
- 2 cups firmly packed baby arugula
- ⅓ cup chopped fresh mint leaves
- 1 cup dried beluga
- 1 clove garlic, minced
- 1 teaspoon minced ginger

Directions

1. Preheat the oven to 400°F.
2. Align a baking sheet with parchment paper.
3. Place the carrots in a large bowl.
4. Drizzle with the oil and maple syrup.
5. Sprinkle with cumin, let toss to coat.
6. Move to the lined baking sheet make sure to spread in a single layer.
7. Season salt and pepper.
8. Let bake for 30 – 40 minutes till brown.
9. Place the lentils in a pot of water to cover by 4 inches.
10. Boil, reduce the heat let simmer for 20 – 30 minutes.
11. Drain excess water.
12. Place in carrots with lentils in a large bowl let settle for 10 minutes.
13. Add arugula, onion, and mint.
14. Combine the remaining ingredients in a small bowl whisk to coat.
15. Pour the dressing over the salad toss to combined.
16. Taste and season accordingly.
17. Drizzle with pomegranate molasses.
18. Serve and enjoy

Roasted and raw carrot salad with avocado

This recipe reflects the power embedded within herbs.

As a result, the carrots are herbed with avocado and mustard dressing.

Very delicious for any meal, lunch or dinner.

Ingredients

- Freshly ground black pepper
- 2 tablespoons of extra-virgin olive oil
- Pinch of red pepper flakes
- Salt
- ⅓ cup of torn fresh leafy herbs
- 1 large ripe avocado
- 4 tablespoons of sunshine salad dressing
- ¾ teaspoon of flaky sea salt
- ⅓ cup of chopped green onion
- 2 pounds of carrots

Directions

1. Preheat your oven to 425 °F.
2. Align a large baking sheet with parchment paper.
3. Toss the carrots on the baking sheet with enough olive oil to coat.
4. Let bake for 25 – 30 minutes until tender and deeply golden on the edges.
5. Place carrot rounds in a bowl filled with water along with a handful of ice cubes. Set aside.
6. After roasting carrots, organize them across a platter.
7. Drain carrots, sprinkle over the roasted carrots.
8. Cut avocado slice half of the avocado, scoop out with a large spoon.
9. Arrange over the salad.
10. Drizzle the salad dressing lightly across the salad.
11. Sprinkle onion and leafy herbs on top.
12. Sprinkle with salt, red pepper flakes.
13. Serve and enjoy.

Orange orzo salad with almond, olives, and feta

This particular recipe features wonderfully bright Mediterranean Sea diet flavors.

It is prepared with toasted almond, parsley, cucumber and green onions among others listed below.

Ingredients

- ¼ cup of fresh-squeezed orange juice
- ½ cup of raw almonds
- 2 tablespoons of white wine vinegar
- 1 cup of chopped flat-leaf parsley
- ¼ teaspoon of salt
- ¼ cup of extra-virgin olive oil
- 1 medium clove garlic, minced
- ½ cup of pitted Kalamata olives
- ½ cup of chopped green onion
- 8 ounces of whole wheat orzo pasta
- Freshly ground black pepper
- ½ cup of raisins, preferably golden
- ½ cup of crumbled feta cheese
- 1 teaspoon of orange zest

Directions

1. Boil salted water in a large pot.
2. Add the orzo let cook according to the package Directions.
3. Drain and reserve some pasta cooking water.
4. Rinse under running water until the orzo cool.
5. In a medium skillet over medium heat, toast the almonds keep stirring to attain fragrance and golden color in 5 minutes.
6. Move almonds to a cutting board, chop.
7. Combine orzo, parsley, chopped almonds, green onion, olives, raisins, and feta in a large bowl.
8. Combine orange zest, garlic, olive oil, orange juice, vinegar, and salt in small cup.
9. Add ¼ cup of the reserved pasta cooking water, whisk to blended.
10. Pour the dressing over the salad, toss to combine.
11. Season with pepper accordingly.
12. Allow orzo salad rest for 10 minutes or more.
13. Again season to taste.
14. Serve an enjoy.

Crunchy Thai peanut quinoa salad

Ingredients

- ½ cup chopped cilantro
- ¼ cup thinly sliced green onion
- 1 teaspoon toasted sesame oil
- 1 ½ cups water
- Pinch of red pepper flakes
- ¼ cup roasted and salted peanuts
- 1 teaspoon grated fresh ginger
- ½ lime, juiced
- ¼ cup smooth peanut butter
- ¾ cup uncooked quinoa
- 3 tablespoons tamari
- 1 tablespoon maple syrup
- 1 tablespoon rice vinegar
- 1 cup grated carrot
- 1 cup thinly sliced snow peas
- 2 cups shredded cabbage

Directions

1. In a medium-sized pot, combine quinoa and water.

2. Boil over medium heat, then reduce lower the heat to simmer all the water is absorbed.
3. Take off heat source, cover let sit for 5 minutes. Set aside.
4. Whisk the peanut butter and tamari till smooth.
5. Add and whisk the remaining ingredients until smooth. Add water if too thick.
6. In a large serving bowl, combine the quinoa, carrot, cilantro, shredded cabbage, snow peas, and green onion, toss.
7. Introduce peanut sauce, toss again until fully coated.
8. Taste and season accordingly.
9. Garnish with peanut.
10. Serve and enjoy.

Colorful veggie lettuce wraps

This recipe is largely a healthy delicious appetizer or just a light meal.

It is vegan with colorful wraps.

Ingredients

- 2 tablespoons of tamari
- 2 heads of butter lettuce
- 3 cups of thinly sliced crisp vegetables
- 2 teaspoons of toasted sesame oil
- ¼ teaspoon of salt
- 4 ½ ounces of soba noodles
- ¾ cup of sliced green onions
- 1 ½ cups of edamame hummus
- ¼ cup of rice vinegar
- 2 tablespoons of sesame seeds

Directions

1. Bring a pot of salted water to boil.
2. In a medium sized bowl, combine vinegar, vegetables, and salt, toss to combine, then let mixture marinate for 10 minutes.

3. Cook the soba noodles as per package instruction.
4. Drain, then return them to the pot, place in stir in sesame seeds, onions, tamari, and sesame oil. Set aside.
5. Spread hummus over the center of a lettuce leaf.
6. Top with bit of soba noodles, pickled veggies.
7. Sprinkle lightly with sesame seeds
8. Serve and enjoy.

Chicken bacon salad with honey mustard dressing

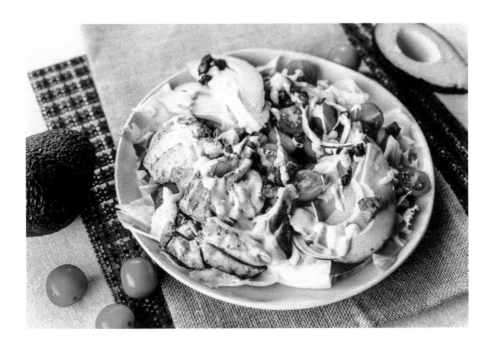

With a juicy chicken breast, this is a quick easy recipe to make in 20 minutes.

The crispy bacon is made together with veggies suitable for vegetarians as the Mediterranean Sea diet agitates.

It is a perfect tasty meal for the day, do not miss to try it out with the step by step procedure below.

Ingredients

- Salt & black pepper
- 2 teaspoon of extra virgin olive oil
- ½ small onion, optional
- 4 teaspoon of white wine vinegar
- 1 cup cherry tomatoes
- 8 ounces thin-sliced chicken breasts
- 2 tablespoons of honey
- 2 tablespoons of lemon juice
- ⅓ cup parmesan cheese, grated
- 6 tablespoons of extra virgin olive oil
- 5 ounces of mixed lettuce leaves
- 2 teaspoon of spicy mustard
- Paprika

Directions

1. Fry the bacon in a frying pan.
2. Move it onto a plate lined with paper kitchen towel when it is ready fried to get rid of the excess fat.
3. Clean the pan of any excess fat then add in the olive oil.
4. Season the chicken breasts with salt, pepper and paprika on every side.
5. Cook on both sides for 4 minutes or till when ready cooked.

6. Cut the cherry tomatoes in halves and slice the onion into rings.
7. Divide mixed onion, lettuce leaves, cherry tomatoes in two separate bowls.
8. Top with chicken slices, parmesan and bacon.
9. Serve and enjoy.

Dad's Greek salad

Salads are a healthy sauce of diet regardless which salad.

The dad's Greek salad is distinctive because of the olives, feta, cucumber and tomatoes.

The olive oil is used to dress the salad with some vinegar and cheese as indicated below.

Ingredients

- 3 tablespoons of red wine vinegar
- ¼ cup of olive oil
- 4 large tomatoes coarsely cup and seeds removed
- 2 cups of thinly sliced cucumbers
- A small red onion cut into two and thinly sliced
- ¼ teaspoon of salt
- 1/8 teaspoon of pepper
- ¼ teaspoon of dried oregano (this is option)
- ¾ cup of pitted Greek olives
- ¾ cup of crumbled feta cheese

Directions

1. Place all the cucumbers, onion, tomatoes in one large bowl at once.

2. Get a small bowl to whisk oil, vinegar, pepper, oregano, and salt

3. Blend until it is finely blended.

4. Drizzle over salad and toast it to coat.

5. Then fill the top with olives and cheese

6. Serve and enjoy

Tzatziki potato salad

Ingredients

- 2 tablespoons snipped fresh dill
- 1 carton (12 ounces) refrigerated tzatziki sauce
- 2 celery ribs, thinly sliced
- 2 tablespoons minced fresh parsley
- ¼ teaspoon celery salt
- 3 pounds small red potatoes, halved
- 2 green onions, chopped
- ½ cup plain Greek yogurt
- ¼ teaspoon pepper
- ½ teaspoon salt
- 1 tablespoon minced fresh mint, optional

Directions

1. Place the potatoes in an oven; preferably a Dutch oven.
2. Cover the potatoes with water then bring to boil.
3. Continue to cook over reduced heat for about 10 – 15 minutes until tender.
4. Drain the excess water and cool completely.
5. Mix the tzatziki sauce, yogurt, celery, dill, parsley, salt, green onions, pepper, and celery salt in a smaller bowl.
6. Spoon over the cooked potatoes then toss to coat.

7. Refrigerate while covered until cold.

8. Serve and enjoy

Mediterranean cobb salad

The Mediterranean cobb salad are classic diet, mainly when there is a flair added to it.

The ingredients and instruction are listed below.

Ingredients

- ½ cup of sour cream or plain yogurt
- ¼ cup of milk
- 1 package of falafel mix (6 ounces)
- ¼ cup of chopped seeded peeled cucumber
- ½ cup of pitted finely chopped Greek olives
- 8 cups of bacon strips, cooked and crumbled
- 2 medium sized finely seeded and chopped tomatoes
- 1 medium ripe peeled and chopped avocado
- 3 hard boiled large chopped eggs
- 4 cups of baby spinach
- 4 cups of torn romaine
- ¼ teaspoon of salt
- 1 teaspoon of minced parsley

Directions

1. Cook the falafel depending on the manufacturer's Directions.
2. Let it cool off
3. Crumble and or coarsely chop falafel
4. Combine the sour cream, cucumber, parsley, salt and milk in a small bowl
5. In a separate larger bowl, combine spinach and romaine.
6. Transfer to a platter
7. Organize the crumbled falafel and the remaining ingredients over greens
8. Drizzle with dressing ready for serving

Nectarine and beet salad

This recipe makes a scrumptious inclusion to variety of mixed greens mainly with the beets, nectarines and feta cheese.

The choice of ingredients may not reflect your favorite salad but that is a lie of one's eyes.

This salad can become your favorite choice for a home salad.

Ingredients

- ½ cup of crumbled feta cheese
- ½ of medium sized sliced nectarines
- 1 can of sliced drained beets (14 – ½ ounces)
- 2 packages of spring greens mixed salad (5 ounces each)
- ½ cup of balsamic vinaigrette

Directions

1. Toss all greens in a serving dish with nectarine and vinaigrette
2. Top with cheese and the beets
3. Serve immediately for a better taste

Balsamic cucumber salad

Cucumber is a perfect healthy salad for variety of dishes especially for kabobs, chicken and or anything hot off the grill.

The Directions and directions are shown below.

Ingredients

- ½ cup of balsamic vinaigrette
- 1 medium halved and thinly sliced red onions
- 1 large halved and sliced cucumber
- 2 cups of grape tomatoes cut into half

Directions

1. Combine the tomatoes, onions, cucumber in a large bowl
2. Introduce vinaigrette then toss to coat.
3. Refrigerate when it is cover until serving
4. Stir in the cheese and then serve with a slotted spoon
5. Enjoy

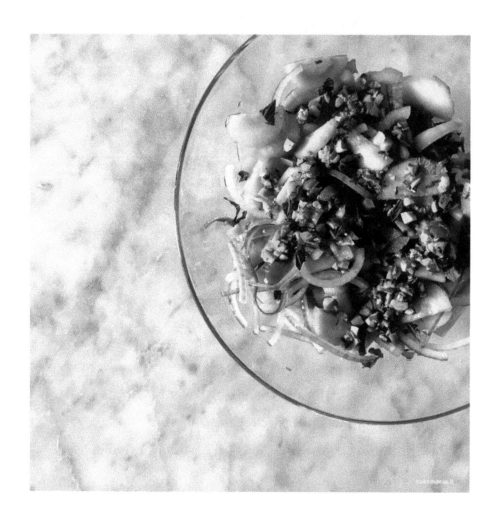

Tzatziki shrimp cucumber rounds

Ingredients

- 2 tablespoons of finely chopped peeled cucumber
- 2 medium size cucumbers slices cut into ¼ -in
- 1.4 cup of reduced fat plain yogurt
- 1/8 teaspoon of garlic salt
- 6 bacon strips
- 1/8 teaspoon of dill weed
- 1 or 2 tablespoons of canola oil
- 24 shrimp peeled and deveined (32 – 40 pound)

Instruction

1. Combine the yogurt, garlic salt, dill and chopped cucumber to set aside in a small bowl.
2. Lengthwise and widthwise, evenly cut each bacon in halves.
3. Using the bacon, wrap each piece of shrimp and lock them with a toothpick.
4. In a larger nonstick skillet, heat the oil with medium temperature.

5. Cook the shrimp in manageable batches for 3 – 4 minutes on every side until crispy
6. Spoon the yogurt sauce on each cucumber slice.
7. Top with the shrimp
8. Serve and enjoy

Tomato feta salad

This recipe is perfect for balsamic dressing.

It can be topped and served with a variety of dishes or even combined with other veggies to quench the appetite for fresh healthy vegetables.

Below are the ingredients and Directions.

Ingredients

- 2 tablespoons of balsamic vinegar
- ¼ cup of crumbles feta cheese
- 1 – ¼ teaspoon of minced basil (fresh or dried)
- ½ teaspoon of salt
- ½ cup of coarsely chopped sweet onions
- 1 pound of grape or cherry tomatoes
- 2 tablespoon of olive oil

Directions

1. Using a larger bowl, combine the basil, salt, and vinegar.
2. Introduce the onion then toss to coat.
3. Let it settle for 5 minutes.

4. Introduce the tomatoes, feta cheese, and oil and toss to coat.
5. Serve and enjoy

Cherry tomato salad

This very recipe emerged from the need and urgency to use bumper crops of delicious cherry tomatoes commonly grown.

Since then, the ingredients and directions below have been used to utilize cherry tomatoes.

Ingredients

- 1 or 2 teaspoons of minced oregano
- ¼ cup of canola oil
- ¼ cup of minced parsley
- ½ teaspoon of salt
- ½ teaspoon of sugar
- 1 quart of cherry tomatoes
- 3 tablespoons of white vinegar
- 1 teaspoon of minced basil

Directions

1. In a shallow bowl, place all the tomatoes.
2. In another small bowl, mix whisk oil, salt, sugar, and vinegar until evenly blended.
3. Stir in the herbs.
4. Pour the over tomatoes gently to toss and coat.

5. Cover and refrigerate overnight.
6. Serve and enjoy

Greek salad dressing

Ingredients

- ½ teaspoon of dried oregano
- ¼ teaspoon of pepper
- ½ cup of olive oil
- ½ teaspoon of salt
- ¼ cup of red wine vinegar
- 2 minced garlic cloves
- 1 teaspoon of Dijon mustard
- 2 teaspoons of lemon juice

Directions

1. In a tight fitting lid jar, combine all the ingredients at once.
2. Shake well until fully blended.
3. Serve and enjoy.

Garden tomato salad

One can make this garden tomato recipe conveniently at any time as long as they have a garden of fresh tomatoes.

The nourishing looks of a fresh tomato makes this a perfect salad for a Mediterranean Sea diet.

Ingredients

- ¼ cup of olive oil
- ½ teaspoon of salt
- 2 tablespoons of cider vinegar
- 1 minced garlic clove
- 1 teaspoon of minced chives
- 1 teaspoon of minced basil
- 1 large sweet onions cut into wedges
- 3 large tomatoes cut into wedges
- 1 large sliced cucumber

Directions

1. Combine cucumber, tomatoes, and onions in a large bowl.

2. In another small bowl, whisk the dressing ingredients until uniformly blended (the remaining ingredients apart from tomatoes, cucumber, and onions)

3. Drizzle over the salad then slowly toss to coat.

4. Serve immediately or store under refrigeration if need be.

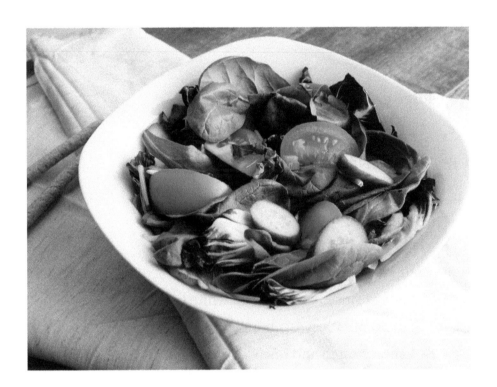

White bean salad

This recipe includes the preparation of white beans loaded with Mediterranean Sea diet flavors.

Unlike other recipes, this one does not involve fancy dressing; as such, it is only lemon juice and extra virgin oil that is important.

Ingredients

- 1 cup chopped fresh parsley
- 4 green onions, chopped
- 1 English cucumber, diced
- 10 orzo grape or cherry tomatoes, halved
- Feta cheese, optional
- Salt and pepper
- 2 cans of rinsed and drained white beans
- 15 to 20 mint leaves, chopped
- 1 lemon, zested and juiced
- Extra virgin olive oil
- 1 teaspoon of Za'atar
- ½ teaspoon of Sumac and Aleppo .

Directions

1. In a large bowl, combine the tomatoes, green onions, mint, cucumber, beans, and parsley.
2. Proceed to add lemon zest.
3. Season with pepper and salt.
4. Add the za'atar, Aleppo pepper, and sumac.
5. Finish up the recipe with lemon juice which can be drizzled with 2 or 3 tablespoon of extra virgin olive oil.
6. Do a thorough toss to let combine.
7. Adjust the season according to the taste.
8. Introduce the feta cheese, if desired.
9. Allow the salad to settle in the dressing for 30 – 31 minutes just before serving
10. Serve.

3-ingredient Mediterranean salad

Ingredients

- 1 teaspoon of ground Sumac
- salt
- 2 teaspoons of freshly squeezed lemon juice
- 1 Large diced cucumber
- ½ to ¾ packed cup/ 15 to 20 g chopped fresh parsley leaves
- ½ teaspoon of black pepper
- 2 teaspoon of Early Harvest extra virgin olive oil
- 6 diced Roma tomatoes

Directions

1. Put the diced tomatoes, parsley in a larger salad bowl.
2. Add salt and set aside for approximately 4 minutes
3. Add all remaining ingredients and toss the salad gently.
4. Give the flavors some minutes to melt before serving.
5. Enjoy

Coconut quinoa and kale with tropical pesto

Ingredients

- Salt and freshly ground black pepper, to taste
- 1 cup of quinoa, rinsed
- ½ cup of olive oil
- 1 cup of light coconut milk
- ½ lime, juiced
- 4 cloves garlic
- 1 small bunch of kale
- ⅓ cup of chopped red onion
- pinch red pepper flakes
- ⅓ cup of large, unsweetened coconut flakes
- 2 cups of cilantro, packed
- Scant ½ cup of raw, unsalted cashews

Directions

1. Combine coconut milk with water in a medium sized saucepan, bring to a boil.
2. Add the quinoa, and simmer covered for 17 minutes, until the water is absorbed.

3. Remove, fluff with a fork and mix in the red onion. Set aside.
4. Combine cilantro together with the cashews and garlic in a food processor.
5. Processing the mixture as you slowly drizzle in the olive oil.
6. Season with salt, pepper, lime juice and red pepper flakes, and blend well.
7. In a medium serving bowl, combine the warm coconut quinoa, chopped kale and pesto.
8. Mix well with a big spoon.
9. Taste, and adjust the seasoning
10. In a skillet over medium heat, toast the coconut flakes briefly until golden, stirring often.
11. Serve and enjoy topped with coconut flakes.

Stacked tomato, summer vegetable, and grilled bread salad

The stacked tomato, summer vegetable recipe is a great Mediterranean Sea diet with an array of vegetables and herbs which are beautifully grilled.

Ingredients

- Thick slices of whole wheat peasant bread
- 1 cup of sliced cherry tomatoes
- 4 tablespoons of olive oil
- 2 tablespoons of finely chopped and drained oil-packed sun-dried tomatoes
- Sea salt
- 1 tablespoon of red wine vinegar
- 3 cups of baby arugula leaves
- 1 tablespoon of lemon juice
- 1 tablespoon of chopped fresh mint and basil
- 4 ounces of goat cheese
- 2 large zucchini
- 1 teaspoon of honey
- ½ teaspoon of finely chopped Kalamata olives

- 2 red bell peppers
- ½ teaspoon of minced fresh garlic
- ¼ teaspoon of ground sea salt

Directions

1. In a small bowl, whisk olive oil, sundried tomatoes, red wine vinegar, lemon juice, mint and basil, honey, Kalamata olives, garlic, and sea salt.
2. Fold in the tomatoes, let rest.
3. Hold red bell peppers directly over the flame of a gas stove, until the peppers are blackened.
4. Transfer the peppers to a bowl and cover tightly, let cool for 20 minutes, and peel, and cut.
5. Reduce the grill heat to medium.
6. Brush zucchini slices on both sides with olive oil and sprinkle with salt.
7. Brush slices of bread with olive oil on both sides and sprinkle with salt.
8. Arrange the bread slices and zucchini pieces in a single layer on the grill and close the lid.
9. Let until golden brown on both sides. Meanwhile cook the zucchini until well-marked on the first side for 5 minutes, then flip and cook the same way.
10. Transfer the zucchini to a plate and cover loosely to retain heat.

11. Rub the grilled bread on both sides with the garlic clove.
12. Serve and enjoy sprinkled with herbs and scattered lettuce leaves.

Sweet corn salad wraps

Ingredients

- 6 ears of fresh corn, kernels removed
- 1 small red onion, chopped finely
- ½ red bell pepper, chopped
- Handful of cherry tomatoes
- ½ cup of chopped fresh cilantro
- 1 teaspoon of ancho chili powder
- pinch of cayenne pepper
- 2 small limes, juiced
- Sea salt and black pepper
- 1 teaspoon of olive oil
- 1 head of white cabbage
- 2 small corn tortillas
- 1 avocado

Directions

1. Start by combining the raw corn kernels together with the onion, cherry tomatoes, cilantro, bell pepper, chili powder, cayenne pepper, and the juice of limes in a mixing bowl.
2. Season with salt and pepper.
3. Place each leaf of cabbage on its own in a small plate.

4. In a small skillet, on medium-high heat, pour in enough oil to form a thin film on the surface.

5. Then, add the tortilla strips, sprinkled with bit of salt, let fry until crisp, stirring occasionally.

6. Remove tortilla strips from skillet and drain.

7. Spoon about ½ cup of the salsa mixture onto each leaf, then top with crispy tortilla strips and avocado.

8. Serve and enjoy immediately.

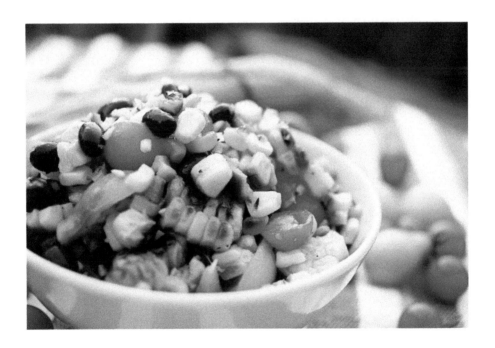

Raw kale salad with creamy tahini dressing

Ingredients

- Dash of tamari or soy sauce
- 1 bunch of curly kale
- Sea salt
- Big pinch red pepper flakes
- ⅓ cup of water
- 1 avocado
- 6 carrots
- Small handful of chopped cilantro
- 2 teaspoons of sesame seeds
- ¼ cup tahini
- 1 tablespoon of white miso
- 1 ½ tablespoons of rice vinegar
- ½ teaspoon toasted sesame oil

Directions

1. Sprinkle a small pinch of sea salt over the prepared kale and massage the leaves briefly.

2. In a small bowl, whisk together the tahini, white miso, rice vinegar, sesame oil, red pepper flakes, water, and tamari.

3. Divide the kale into two bowls, drizzle in the salad dressing, toss thoroughly.

4. Top the salad with carrot ribbons, diced avocado, and some chopped carrot greens.

5. Serve and enjoy.

Saladu nebbe

Ingredients

- 2 serrano peppers or 1 habanero
- ¼ cup of fresh lime juice
- 1 cup of chopped parsley
- 1 medium cucumber, seeded and finely chopped
- Sliced avocado
- ½ cup of olive oil
- 5 cups of cooked black-eyed peas
- Cooked brown basmati rice
- 10 scallions, roughly chopped
- 1 red bell pepper, stemmed, seeded, and finely chopped
- 1 cup cherry, chopped
- Sea salt and freshly ground black pepper, to taste

Directions

1. In a large bowl, whisk together the lime juice with the parsley.
2. Keep whisking as you drizzle in the olive oil to make a smooth dressing.

3. Add the black-eyed peas together with the scallions, bell pepper, tomato, cucumber, and minced pepper to the bowl.
4. Season the mixture with salt and pepper, toss the salad.
5. Pack well and refrigerate overnight for a better taste.
6. Serve and enjoy on top of cooked brown basmati rice topped with avocado slices.

Wheat berries

Ingredients

- ½ teaspoon of ground sea salt
- 1 cup of dried wheat berries
- ¼ teaspoon of red pepper flakes
- 2 cups of cooked chickpeas
- 4 carrots
- 1 small lemon, juiced
- ⅓ cup of olive oil
- Ground black pepper, to taste
- ½ cup of feta cheese, crumbled
- 6 cups of arugula
- 2 teaspoons of honey
- 2 garlic cloves, pressed

Directions

1. Bring 4 quarts of water to a boil in a large pot.
2. Stir in the wheat berries with salt.
3. Cover the pot halfway, let cook, stirring often, until the berries are tender.
4. Drain the wheat berries, let cool to room temperature.
5. Then, whisk olive oil together with the honey, garlic, red pepper flakes, lemon juice, sea salt, and black pepper.

6. Transfer the cooled wheat berries to a big bowl.

7. Add the chickpeas together with the carrots, feta cheese, and arugula, toss to combine.

8. Drizzle in the dressing and toss to coat.

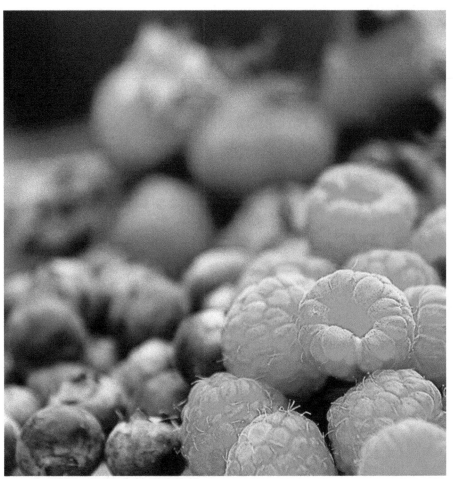

9. Serve and enjoy warm.

Ribboned asparagus and quinoa salad

Ingredients

- 2 tablespoons of pine nuts
- 1 cup of cooked quinoa
- 7 stalks of asparagus
- 2 ounces of Parmesan, shaved
- Black pepper, to taste
- 1 small lemon
- olive oil
- Sea salt, to taste

Directions

1. Combine rinsed quinoa with enough water in a saucepan.
2. Bring to a boil, cover and reduce heat to a simmer.
3. Let cook for 15 minutes to absorbed all the water.
4. In a skillet over medium heat, stirring often, toast the pine nut for 10 minutes.
5. In a bowl, combine cooked quinoa together with the shaved asparagus.
6. Squeeze in most of the juice of half a lemon.
7. Drizzle with olive oil.

8. Sprinkle with sea salt and ground black pepper, toss to coat.
9. Sprinkle with the pine nuts.
10. Serve and enjoy.

Watercress and forbidden rice salad with ginger vinaigrette

Ingredients

- 3 stalks of celery, thinly sliced
- 1-inch nub of ginger, grated or finely chopped
- ¼ cup of green onion, chopped
- 3 cloves garlic, pressed
- 2 tablespoons of rice wine vinegar
- 1 ½ cups of cooked forbidden rice
- 1 yellow bell pepper, chopped
- ¼ cup of peanut oil, olive oil
- 2 teaspoons of toasted sesame oil
- 2 ½ teaspoons of reduced-sodium tamari
- 1 ½ cups of shelled edamame
- ½ teaspoon of agave nectar
- Pinch red pepper flakes
- 1 big bunch watercress

Directions

1. Whisk ginger, garlic, rice wine vinegar, peanut oil, sesame oil, tamari, agave nectar, and red pepper flakes all together, set aside.

2. Cook rice as instructed on the package.
3. Bring a pot of water to a boil and pour in frozen edamame.
4. Lower the heat to a simmer and cook until the edamame is warmed through in just 5 minutes.
5. Drain, set aside to cool.
6. Toss all of the prepared produce in a big bowl.
7. Once the edamame and rice have cooled, add them to the bowl and toss.
8. Serve and enjoy chilled.

Apple slaw for winter

This Mediterranean Sea diet apple recipe features a crunchy cabbage, tasty for any fruit or even vegetable lover for a breakfast.

Ingredients

- 2 medium apples
- Scant ¼ cup of olive oil
- ½ cup chopped cilantro
- 2 teaspoons of Dijon mustard
- 1 tablespoon of honey
- 1 lime, juiced
- Sea salt and pepper, to taste
- 1 small purple cabbage
- 8 radishes, stems and ends removed

Directions

1. In a big bowl, whisk together olive oil with mustard, honey and lime juice.
2. Toss the chopped cabbage, radish, and apple into the bowl.

3. Toss the chopped ingredients with the dressing using a hand.
4. Then, add salt and pepper, to taste.
5. Cover and refrigerate for an hour.
6. Mix in the chopped cilantro.
7. Serve and enjoy immediately.

Cucumber dill salad

This a perfectly refreshing Mediterranean Sea diet recipe on its own as a standalone, yet incredibly tasty drawing its flavor from garlic, onions and herbs.

Ingredients

- ½ cup of crumbled feta cheese
- 1 teaspoon of minced garlic
- 3 cucumbers, seeded and chopped
- 1 red onion, chopped
- Salt and pepper, to taste
- ⅓ cup of finely chopped fresh dill
- 1 lime, juiced
- 3 tomatoes, seeded and chopped
- 3 tablespoons of white wine vinegar
- ¼ cup of olive oil

Directions

1. In a large bowl, toss all of the ingredients together.
2. Season with salt and pepper.
3. Refrigerate for hours to circulate in the flavors.
4. Serve and enjoy.

Vegan sour cream

If you are a vegan having challenges in identifying a recipe that suits your taste and preference, then look no further.

Vegan sour cream is gluten free and it features herbs, vegetables and fruits.

Ingredients

- ¼ teaspoon of Dijon mustard
- ½ cup of water
- Heaping ¼ teaspoon of fine sea salt
- 1 cup of raw cashews
- 1 tablespoon of lemon juice
- 1 teaspoon of apple cider vinegar

Directions

1. In a blender, combine the cashews together with water, lemon juice, vinegar, salt, and mustard.
2. Blend until the mixture is smooth and creamy.
3. Taste, and adjust the seasoning accordingly to your preference.
4. Serve and enjoy immediately or chill the sour cream for later.

Arugula, apples, and Manchego in cider vinaigrette recipe

This is a Spanish Mediterranean diet style.

It blends peppery arugula, juicy apples, Manchego with crunchy almonds then tossed in a cider vinaigrette.

Ingredients

- 1 teaspoon of Dijon mustard
- 1/4 teaspoon of ground black pepper
- 1 crisp apple
- 3 1/2 ounces of Manchego, thinly sliced
- 1/2 cup of sliced almonds
- 2 tablespoons of cider vinegar
- Heaping 1/4 teaspoon of salt
- 6 tablespoons of vegetable oil
- 5 ounces of arugula
- 2 teaspoons of maple syrup
- 1 tablespoon of chopped shallots

Directions

1. Begin by whisking cider vinegar, vegetable oil, maple syrup, Dijon mustard, shallots, salt and ground black pepper in a small bowl. Set aside.
2. Place arugula in serving bowl.
3. Whisk the vinaigrette again until well combined, add the salad, little by little, until greens are well dressed.
4. Slice the apple and toss into salad with Manchego and almonds.
5. Taste and adjust seasoning.
6. Serve and enjoy.

Healthy apple muffins

Ingredients

- ½ cup of plain Greek yogurt
- 1 ¾ cups of white whole wheat flour
- ½ cup of applesauce
- 1 ½ teaspoons of baking powder
- 1 teaspoon of vanilla extract
- 1 teaspoon of ground cinnamon
- ½ teaspoon of baking soda
- 1 tablespoon of turbinado sugar
- ½ teaspoon of salt
- 1 cup of grated apple
- 1 cup of apple diced into cubes
- ⅓ cup of melted coconut oil
- ½ cup of maple syrup
- 2 eggs

Directions

1. Preheat your oven to 425°F.
2. Grease 12 cups on the muffin tin with butter.
3. In a large mixing bowl, combine the flour together with the baking powder, cinnamon, baking soda, and salt. Blend well.

4. Add the grated apple with chopped apple. Stir to combine.

5. In another separate medium mixing bowl, combine the oil together with maple syrup and whisk.

6. Add the eggs and beat well.

7. Add the yogurt, applesauce, and vanilla, mix well.

8. Mix the wet ingredients with the dry ones, and mix to combined.

9. Sprinkle the tops of the muffins with turbinado sugar.

10. Let bake for 16 minutes, or until the muffins are golden on top.

11. Place the muffin tin on a cooling rack to cool.

12. Serve and enjoy.

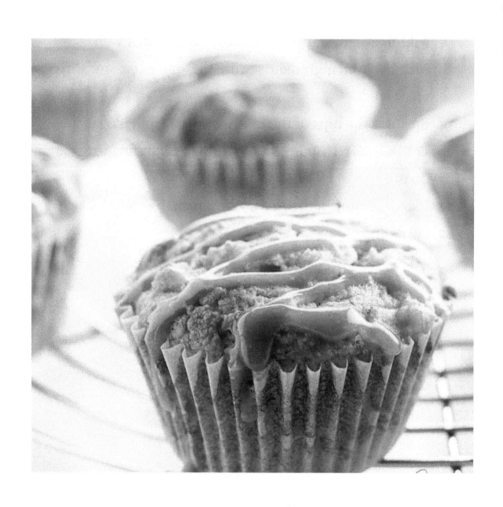

Vibrant orange and arugula salad

Ingredients

- ¼ teaspoon of salt
- 3 tablespoons of lemon juice
- 6 ounces of baby arugula
- 2 oranges, peeled and sliced
- 1 ½ teaspoons of honey
- 2 ounces of goat cheese, crumbled
- Pinch of ground cinnamon
- ¼ cup of extra-virgin olive oil
- ¼ cup of thinly sliced radishes
- ¼ cup of sliced almonds

Directions

1. In a small skillet warm the almonds over medium heat until fragrant in 5 minutes.
2. Transfer to a bowl, let cool.
3. Place the arugula on a large serving platter.
4. Organize the oranges with toasted almonds, goat cheese, and radishes on top.

5. Sprinkle the top lightly with a pinch of cinnamon. Set aside.
6. In a small bowl, combine the olive oil together with the lemon juice, honey, and salt. Whisk to blend.
7. Taste, and adjust the seasoning accordingly.
8. Drizzle the dressing lightly over the salad.
9. Serve and enjoy.

Celery salad with dates, almond, and parmesan

Ingredients

- ¼ cup of extra-virgin olive oil
- 2 ounces of Parmigiano-Reggiano cheese
- ½ cup of raw almonds
- 4 dates, pitted and roughly chopped
- 3 tablespoons of fresh lemon juice
- ¼ teaspoon of red pepper flakes
- Sea salt, to taste
- 8 long celery stalks
- Freshly ground black pepper, to taste

Directions

1. Soak the celery in ice water for about 20 minutes.
2. Drain and pat dry, then pile the celery into a medium serving bowl.
3. Warm the almonds over medium heat, stirring often, until fragrant and toasted for 7 minutes.
4. Transfer to a cutting board and chop.
5. Add the celery leaves to the bowl of celery with chopped almonds, dates, lemon juice, and red pepper flakes.

6. Season with salt and pepper, toss to combine.

7. Add the cheese and olive oil, toss.

8. Serve and enjoy.

Greek wedge salad

The Greek wedge salad takes pride in pilled vegetables on top mainly romaine lettuce, tomatoes, and olives.

This Mediterranean Sea diet is best consumed immediately than later.

Ingredients

- 2 tablespoons of tahini
- 1 ½ cups of cherry tomatoes
- 3 cloves of garlic, minced
- ⅔ cup of cucumber
- ⅔ cup of chopped celery
- ¼ cup of pitted Kalamata olives
- Freshly ground black pepper
- 1 shallot, thinly sliced
- 2 heads of romaine
- ½ teaspoon of grain sea salt
- 1 tablespoon of lemon juice
- Pinch of salt
- ¼ cup of extra virgin olive oil
- 3 tablespoons of lemon juice

Directions

1. In a medium mixing bowl, combine the tomatoes together with the cucumber, olives, shallot, lemon juice, celery, and a pinch of salt. Toss, let marinate.
2. In a small bowl, combine extra virgin olive oil, lemon juice, tahini, garlic, sea salt, and black pepper, whisk.
3. Season generously with pepper, whisk.
4. Place each romaine halve on its own dinner plate.
5. Top with the tomato salad mixture.
6. Drizzle the dressing over the salads
7. Serve and enjoy.

Massaged broccoli rabe salad with sunflower seeds and cranberries

This recipe turns broccoli to a delicious salad after dressing with garlicky and lemony and other herbs and seeds.

Ingredients

- 1 large clove garlic
- 2 bunches of broccoli rabe
- 1 tablespoon of lemon juice
- ¼ cup of sunflower seeds
- ½ teaspoon of Dijon mustard
- ½ cup of chopped celery
- ¼ teaspoon of salt
- ⅓ cup of grated Parmesan cheese
- ¼ cup of dried cranberries
- 3 tablespoons of olive oil

Directions

1. In a medium skillet over medium heat, toast the sunflower seeds for 5 minutes.

2. Remove, and set aside.
3. In a small bowl, whisk together the lemon juice, mustard, olive oil, garlic, and salt until emulsified.
4. Pour the dressing over the leaves and gently massage the dressing into the leaves.
5. Taste, and adjust the seasoning.
6. Add the chopped celery together with the grated Parmesan, toasted sunflower seeds, and dried cranberries to the serving bowl.
7. Serve and enjoy.

Mega crunchy romaine salad with quinoa

Ingredients

- ½ cup of raw sunflower seeds
- ½ teaspoon of grain sea salt
- 1 small head of romaine
- 1 cup of shredded carrots
- ¼ teaspoon of chili powder
- 2 teaspoons of honey
- 1 cup of chopped cabbage
- ½ cup of chopped radishes
- 2 medium cloves garlic
- ½ cup of dried cranberries
- ⅓ cup of olive oil
- ⅔ cup of uncooked quinoa
- 3 tablespoons of lime juice
- 2 tablespoons of rice vinegar
- 1 ⅓ cups of water
- ¼ cup of fresh cilantro

Directions

1. Bring the mixture of quinoa and water to a boil over medium-high heat.
2. Lower the heat, let simmer. Cook until the quinoa has absorbed all of the water.
3. Remove, let the quinoa steam for 5 minutes.
4. Combine the sunflower seeds and olive oil in a medium skillet.
5. Cook, stirring frequently over medium heat, until the seeds are fragrant.
6. Remove, set aside to cool.
7. In a large serving bowl, combine the carrots, cabbage, radishes, prepared romaine, and cranberries.
8. Add quinoa and sunflower seed to the bowl as well.
9. Combine the olive oil, rice vinegar, cilantro, honey, garlic, sea salt, and chili powder, blend in a blender.
10. Serve and enjoy.

Thai mango salad with peanut dressing

Ingredients

- 1 head of butter leaf lettuce
- 1 tablespoon of apple cider vinegar
- 1 teaspoon of sesame oil
- 1 red bell pepper
- 3 ripe champagne mangos, diced
- 2 cloves garlic
- ½ cup of sliced green onion
- ⅓ cup of chopped roasted peanuts
- ¼ cup of chopped fresh cilantro
- 1 tablespoon of honey
- Pinch of red pepper flakes
- 1 medium jalapeño
- ¼ cup of creamy peanut butter
- ¼ cup of lime juice
- 1 tablespoon of tamari

Directions

1. Combine butter leaf lettuce, red bell pepper, mango, onion, roasted peanut, cilantro, and jalapeno in a large serving bowl.

2. Combine peanut butter, lime juice, tamari, apple cider vinegar, honey, sesame, garlic, and pepper flakes in a bowl, and whisk to combine.

3. Drizzle the dressing over the salad, toss to combine.

4. Serve and enjoy.

Crispy apple and kohlrabi salad

Ingredients

- 2 tablespoons of lemon juice
- 1 large Honey crisp apple
- ¼ cup of fresh tarragon leaves
- Flaky sea salt
- 2 small kohlrabies
- 3 tablespoons of toasted sunflower seeds
- Lemon zest, to taste
- 2 tablespoons olive oil

Directions

1. In a large serving bowl, combine the kohlrabi together with the apple matchsticks.
2. Add the cheese with sunflower seeds.
3. Drizzle in bit of olive oil and some lemon juice
4. Sprinkle lightly with salt and black pepper.
5. Toss the salad with your hands.
6. Serve and enjoy.

Sundried tomato, spinach, and quinoa salad

Ingredients

- ½ teaspoon of salt
- 1 cup of quinoa
- ⅓ cup of sun-dried tomatoes
- 1 teaspoon of Dijon mustard
- Pinch of red pepper flakes
- 2 cups of roughly chopped fresh spinach
- ⅓ cup of sliced almonds
- Freshly ground black pepper
- 2 cloves garlic
- ¼ teaspoon of olive oil
- Salt, to taste
- 2 tablespoons of olive oil
- 2 tablespoons of lemon juice

Directions

1. Combine quinoa and 2 cups water in a medium saucepan.
2. Bring the mixture to a boil over medium-high heat.
3. Simmer over low heat, until the quinoa has absorbed all of the water.

4. Remove, let the quinoa rest for 5 minutes.
5. Whisk together the olive oil with lemon juice, garlic, mustard, salt and red pepper flakes.
6. Season with freshly ground black pepper.
7. Warm bit of olive oil over medium heat until shimmering.
8. Add the almonds and a dash of salt, let cook, stirring frequently until golden.
9. Let the almonds cool.
10. Transfer the quinoa to the serving bowl.
11. Drizzle all of the dressing on top, toss to combine.
12. Add the chopped sun-dried tomatoes and spinach.
13. Serve and enjoy.

Berry spinach salad with spicy maple sunflower seeds

Ingredients

- ½ teaspoon of Dijon mustard
- 1 tablespoon of balsamic vinegar
- ⅓ cup of sunflower seeds
- 1 ½ teaspoons of maple syrup
- ⅓ cup of crumbled goat cheese
- Pinch salt
- Salt and pepper
- Dash cayenne
- 5 ounces of baby spinach
- 1 ½ cups of total raspberries
- ½ teaspoon of maple syrup
- 3 tablespoons of olive oil

Directions

1. Warm a small non-stick skillet over medium heat, add the sunflower seeds.
2. When the seeds warm up, pour in the maple syrup, a pinch of salt and a tiny dash of cayenne pepper, toast

while stirring constantly until most of the maple syrup has evaporated in 5 minutes.

3. Transfer the seeds to a plate.

4. In a serving bowl, combine the spinach with the berries, crumbled goat cheese, and sunflower seeds.

5. Whisk olive oil, balsamic vinegar, Dijon mustard, maple syrup, salt and pepper until emulsified.

6. Serve and enjoy.

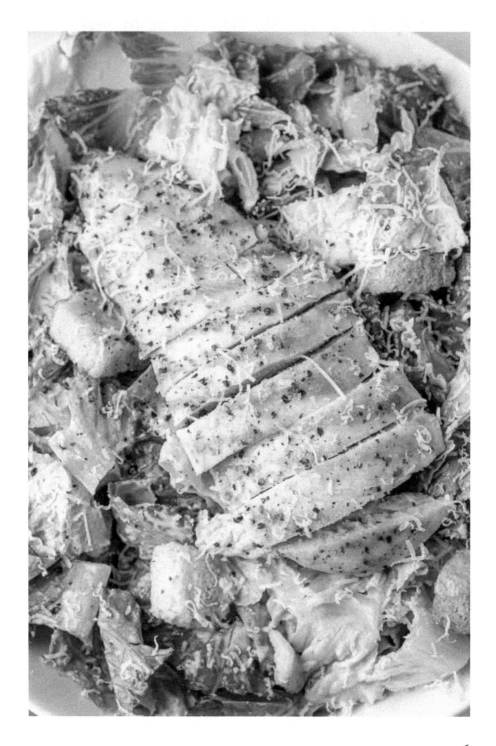